The Comprehensive Alkaline Diet for Beginners and Advanced Users

I0134765

Quick and Easy Recipes to Rebalance your Metabolism and Improve your Energy

Sam Carter

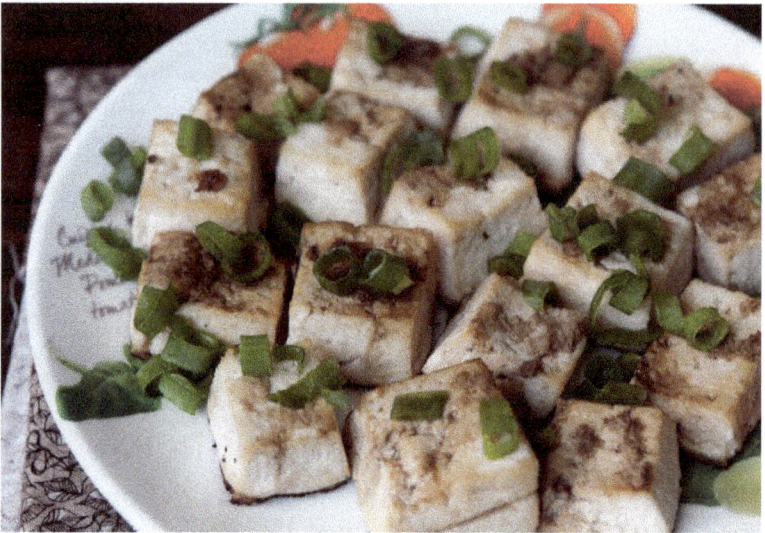

© **Copyright 2021 - All rights reserved.**

The content contained within this book may not be reproduced, duplicated or transmitted without direct written permission from the author or the publisher.

Under no circumstances will any blame or legal responsibility be held against the publisher, or author, for any damages, reparation, or monetary loss due to the information contained within this book. Either directly or indirectly.

Legal Notice:

This book is copyright protected. This book is only for personal use. You cannot amend, distribute, sell, use, quote or paraphrase any part, or the content within this book, without the consent of the author or publisher.

Disclaimer Notice:

Please note the information contained within this document is for educational and entertainment purposes only. All effort has been executed to present accurate, up to date, and reliable, complete information. No warranties of any kind are declared or implied. Readers acknowledge that the author is not engaging in the rendering of legal, financial, medical or professional advice. The content within this book has been derived from various sources. Please consult a licensed professional before attempting any techniques outlined in this book.

By reading this document, the reader agrees that under no circumstances is the author responsible for any losses, direct or indirect, which are incurred as a result of the use of information contained within this document, including, but not limited to, — errors, omissions, or inaccuracies.

Table of Contents

Mushroom, Onion & Brown Rice Sauté

Servings: 2

Total Time: 15 minutes

Ingredients

- 2 tablespoons olive oil, divided
- 2 shallots, thinly sliced
- 2 garlic cloves, minced
- 1 teaspoon ginger, grated
- ¼ teaspoon red chili flakes
- ½ pound crimini mushrooms, sliced
- ½ teaspoon Himalayan salt
- ½ teaspoon black pepper. Crushed
- 1 cup brown rice, cooked
- 1 tablespoon apple cider vinegar
- 1 tablespoon tamari
- 1 tablespoon coconut aminos
- ½ cup arugula
- 1 tablespoon pine nuts, toasted

Directions

1.	Heat oil in a medium skillet over medium heat and add shallots, garlic, ginger and red chili flakes. Cook 3 minutes and then add mushrooms, salt and black pepper.

2.	Cook 8 minutes and then add the rice, vinegar, tamari and coconut aminos. Cook for 2 minutes.

3.	Place arugula in a large bowl and top with mushroom and rice mixture. Garnish with pine nuts and serve immediately.

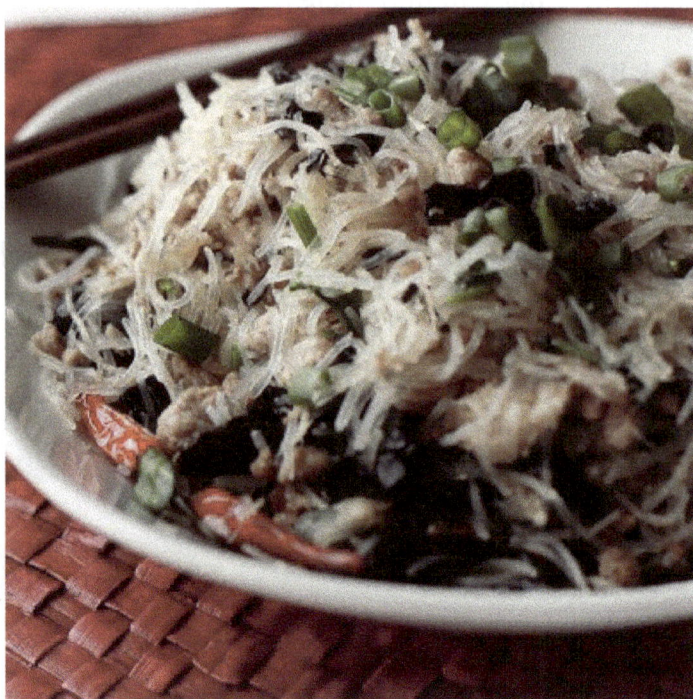

Tofu Ginger Stir-Fry

Servings: 2

Total Time: 25 minutes

Ingredients

- 1 tablespoon sesame oil, divided
- 8 ounces firm tofu, cubed
- 1 garlic clove, minced
- 2 shallots, diced
- 2 tablespoons green onion, sliced
- 1-inch piece ginger, minced
- ¼ teaspoon turmeric
- ½ teaspoon red chili flakes
- 1 tablespoon tamari
- 2 cups Napa cabbage, shredded
- ½ cup fresh shiitake mushrooms
- 1 cup broccoli, cut into florets
- ¼ cup edamame
- 1 zucchini, spiralized into thin noodles
- 1 tablespoon sesame seeds

- 1 tablespoon cilantro, chopped

Directions

1.   Heat half of the oil in a large skillet over medium-high heat. Place tofu and sear on all sides of the cube for a minute each side. Remove tofu from the pan.

2.   Add remaining oil and the garlic, shallot, green onion, ginger, turmeric, red chili flakes and tamari. Cook for 2 minutes, stirring frequently. Add cabbage, mushrooms, broccoli and edamame.

3.   Cook 8-10 minutes or until vegetables are soft. Toss in zucchini noodles and tofu and cook an additional 2 minutes.

4.   Transfer to serving bowl and top with sesame seeds and cilantro.

Cashew Vegetable Skillet

Servings: 2

Total Time: 15 minutes

Ingredients

- 1 tablespoon coconut oil

- ½ red onion, thinly sliced

- 2 garlic cloves, minced

- 1 celery stalk, sliced

- ½ red bell pepper, sliced

- 1 small green chili, seeds removed and diced

- ½ cup raw cashews, toasted

- ½ cup broccoli, cut into florets

- ½ cup cauliflower, cut into florets

- 10 snow pea pods

- 2 tablespoons green onions, sliced

- 1 tablespoon sesame seeds

- 1 tablespoon cilantro, chopped

Sauce

- 1 cup vegetable broth

- 3 tablespoons coconut aminos

- 1 tablespoon tamari

- 1 tablespoon raw honey

- 1 tablespoon sesame oil

- 2 teaspoons apple cider vinegar

- ½ teaspoon red chili flakes

- ½ teaspoon ground ginger

- ⅛ teaspoon ground cloves

- ⅛ teaspoon black pepper, crushed

- 2 teaspoons cornstarch

Directions

1. Make the Sauce by whisking the Sauce ingredients together in a medium bowl until well combined.

2. In a large skillet, heat oil over medium-high heat and sauté the onion, garlic, celery, pepper and chili. After 5 minutes add the cashews, broccoli and cauliflower. Cook 2 minutes and then add the Sauce.

3. Continue cooking for 3 minutes and then add the snow peas. Cook 1 minute.

4.   Transfer to serving bowl and garnish with green onion, sesame seeds and cilantro.

Fried Broccoli Rice

Servings: 2

Total Time: 20 minutes

Ingredients

- 1 tablespoon coconut oil

- 2 shallots, sliced

- 1 small head broccoli, cut into florets

- ½ cup brown rice, cooked and cooled

- 1/3 cup cashews, toasted

- 1 tablespoon green onion, sliced

Sauce

- 2 tablespoons tamari

- 1 tablespoon water

- 1 teaspoon coconut aminos

- 1 teaspoon raw honey

- 1 teaspoon sesame oil

- 1 teaspoon rice wine vinegar

- 1 teaspoon lime juice

- ½ teaspoon red chili flakes

- ½ teaspoon ginger, grated

- 1 garlic clove, minced

- ⅛ teaspoon cloves

Directions

1.   Make the Sauce by whisking the Sauce ingredients together in a medium bowl until well combined.

2.   In a large skillet, heat oil over medium-high heat and sauté the shallot. Cook 5 minutes and then add the broccoli.

3.   Continue cooking for 5 minutes and then add the rice and sauce, making sure to stir well.

4.   Cook 5 minutes and then transfer to serving bowl and garnish with cashews and green onion.

Coconut Lentil Stew

Servings: 2

Total Time: 35 minutes

Ingredients

- 1 tablespoon coconut oil
- ½ teaspoon cumin seeds
- ¼ teaspoon mustard seeds
- ¼ teaspoon fenugreek seeds
- 2 shallots, sliced
- 1-inch piece ginger, grated
- ¼ teaspoon cayenne
- ½ teaspoon ground coriander
- ½ teaspoon ground cumin
- ¼ teaspoon turmeric
- ¼ teaspoon cinnamon
- ½ teaspoon Himalayan salt
- ½ teaspoon black pepper, crushed
- ¾ cup split red lentils
- 1 tomato, diced

- 1 ½ cups water

- ¼ cup coconut milk

- ½ lime, juiced

- 3 cups kale, stems removed and thinly sliced

- 2 tablespoons coconut flakes, toasted

- 2 tablespoons cilantro

Directions

1.   Heat half of the oil in a medium saucepan over medium heat and add the cumin seeds, mustard seeds, fenugreek seeds and shallots. Cook 5 minutes until shallots are soft and spices are fragrant. Add ginger and cook another minute before adding the cayenne, coriander, cumin, turmeric and cinnamon.

2.   Cook spices for 2 minutes and then add the salt, pepper, lentils, tomato and water. Bring to a boil and then reduce heat to low and simmer 10 minutes. Add the coconut milk and lime juice and continue cooking for 10 more minutes.

3.   In a small saucepan, heat remaining coconut oil and quickly sauté the kale, about 5 minutes or until it has wilted.

4.   Transfer mixture from the medium saucepan to a bowl, top with sautéed kale, coconut flakes and cilantro. Serve warm.

Noodle & Pesto Pizza

Servings: 2

Total Time: 30 minutes

Ingredients

- 1 medium sweet potato, spiralized into thin noodles
- 1 tablespoon almond meal
- 1 tablespoon flaxseeds meal
- 1 tablespoon coconut oil
- ¼ teaspoon cumin powder

Pesto

- ½ cup kale
- 1 garlic clove
- 1 tablespoon olive oil
- 1 lemon, juiced
- 1 ½ tablespoons pine nuts
- ¼ teaspoon Himalayan salt
- ¼ teaspoon black pepper, crushed

Topping

- 1 ½ tablespoon olive oil

- 1 ½ cups arugula

- 1 teaspoon lemon juice

- ½ teaspoon oregano

- ¼ teaspoon Himalayan salt

- 1 small tomato, sliced

- ½ small avocado, sliced

Directions

1. Preheat oven to 425°F/220°C.

2. Mix sweet potato, almond meal, flaxseeds meal, coconut oil and cumin together in a medium bowl. Heat a medium, oven-safe skillet over high heat and add the sweet potato mixture, ensuring that it is in a circular shape and pressed down evenly. Cook 5 minutes.

3. Transfer skillet to the oven and cook for 10 minutes.

4. Make the Pesto by adding all the Pesto ingredients to a blender and processing until smooth. Set aside.

5. After 10 minutes, flip sweet potato crust onto a baking tray lined with parchment paper so that the side that had been down in the pan now faces up. Drizzle with the ½ tablespoon of olive oil and place back in the oven for another 10 minutes.

6.   In a small bowl, place the arugula, 1 tablespoon olive oil, lemon juice, oregano and salt. Toss well to coat.

7.   Remove sweet potato crust and spread pesto on top. Arrange tomato and avocado slices in alternating pattern and then top with arugula.

Farmer's Market Salad

Servings: 2

Total Time: 10 minutes

Ingredients

- 1 cup quinoa, cooked
- 2 garlic cloves, minced
- ½ red onion, diced
- ½ bunch kale, stems removed and cut into thin ribbons
- ½ 15 oz. can of white beans, drained and rinsed
- 1 zucchini, grated
- 1 yellow squash, grated
- 1 tomato, diced
- 1/3 cup fresh basil, sliced into ribbons
- 2 tablespoons pumpkin seeds
- 1 lemon, zested and juiced
- 2 tablespoons olive oil
- ½ teaspoon Himalayan salt
- ½ teaspoon black pepper, crushed
- 1 tablespoon parsley, chopped

Directions

1.   In a large bowl, combine all ingredients (except for parsley) and toss well to coat. Let sit 5 minutes so kale softens.

2.   Garnish with parsley before serving.

Kale Chard Warm Salad

Servings: 2

Total Time: 10 minutes

Ingredients

- 2 tablespoons olive oil
- 1 bunch of kale, stems removed and thinly sliced
- 1 bunch of rainbow chard, stems removed and thinly sliced
- 1 cup red cabbage, thinly shredded
- ½ cup sauerkraut
- 1 garlic clove, minced
- ½ lemon, zested and juiced
- ½ teaspoon apple cider vinegar
- ¼ teaspoon Himalayan salt
- ½ teaspoon black pepper, crushed
- 1 cup brown rice, cooked
- 1 tablespoon parsley

Directions

1.   Heat olive oil in a medium skillet over medium-low heat. Add kale, chard, and cabbage and cook 5-7 minutes or until wilted.

2.   Add in sauerkraut, garlic, lemon zest and juice, vinegar, salt and pepper. Cook 1 additional minute.

3.   Serve on top of warm brown rice and garnish with parsley.

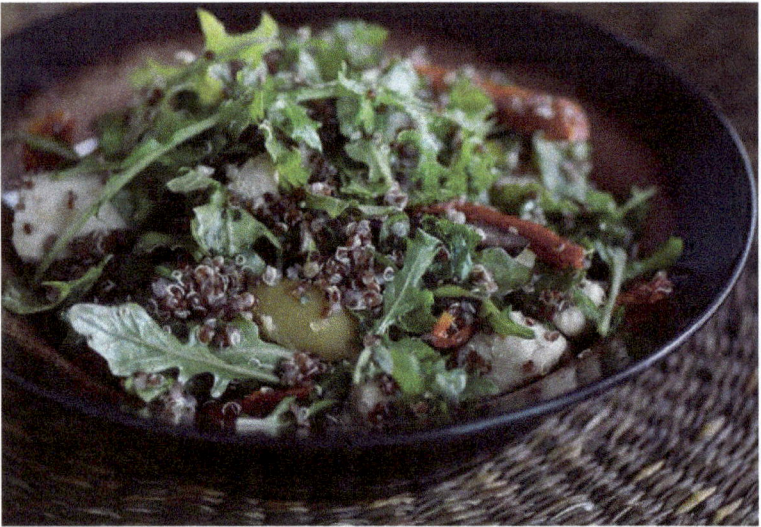

Veggie Medley Skillet

Servings: 2

Total Time: 35 minutes

Ingredients

- 1 small sweet potato
- 3 small eggplants, diced
- 1 cup zucchini, sliced
- 1 teaspoon coconut oil
- 2 garlic cloves, minced
- ½-inch piece ginger, minced
- 2 cups arugula leaves
- 1 lemon, juiced
- 1 teaspoon maple syrup
- ½ teaspoon cayenne pepper
- 1 tomato, diced
- 1 cucumber, sliced
- 1 tablespoon walnuts, crushed
- ½ teaspoon Himalayan salt
- ½ teaspoon black pepper, crushed

Directions

1.   Preheat oven to 350°F/180°C. Poke holes in sweet potato with a fork and rub the eggplant and zucchini with coconut oil. Arrange in sections in a large oven-safe skillet (such as a cast iron pan). Sprinkle with garlic and ginger.

2.   Roast in the oven for 30 minutes or until vegetables are soft.

3.   While vegetables are roasting, combine the arugula, lemon juice, maple syrup, cayenne, tomato, cucumber, walnuts, salt and pepper in a large bowl and toss well to coat.

4.   After 30 minutes, remove skillet from the oven and top with arugula mixture.

5.   Serve from the skillet.

Indian Onion & Peppers

Servings: 2

Total Time: 20 minutes

Ingredients

- 1 ½ tablespoons coconut oil
- 1 medium yellow onion, chopped
- 1 small shallot, sliced
- ½ green bell pepper, chopped
- ½ red bell pepper, chopped
- 2 garlic cloves, chopped
- 1 green chili, chopped
- 1-inch piece ginger, grated
- 1 teaspoon cumin seeds
- ½ teaspoon turmeric powder
- 1 tablespoon cashews
- 3 tablespoons tomato paste
- ½ cup diced tomatoes
- ½ teaspoon garam masala powder
- 1 teaspoon red chili powder

- ½ teaspoon cayenne pepper
- ½ teaspoon Himalayan salt
- 1 tablespoon cilantro, chopped

Directions

1.   Heat coconut oil in a medium pot over medium-high heat. Add the onion, shallot, bell peppers, garlic, chili and ginger. Cook for 8 minutes, stirring occasionally, and then add the cumin seeds, turmeric and cashews.

2.   Cook another 3 minutes before adding the tomato paste, diced tomatoes, garam masala, chili powder, cayenne pepper and salt.

3.   Cook 5 more minutes and remove from heat.

4.   Garnish with cilantro and serve.

Broccoli Pasta

Servings: 2

Total Time: 30 minutes

Ingredients

- 1 small head of broccoli, cut into florets
- 1 ½ tablespoons coconut oil
- 1 garlic clove, minced
- 1 zucchini, spiralized into noodles
- ½ teaspoon red pepper flakes
- ½ yellow onion, thinly sliced
- 1 tablespoon parsley, chopped
- 1 cup lentils, cooked
- ½ teaspoon Himalayan salt
- ½ teaspoon black pepper, crushed
- 1 tablespoon nutritional yeast

Directions

1.   Preheat oven to 400°F/205°C. Line a baking tray with parchment paper. In a medium bowl, toss broccoli with the ½

tablespoon coconut oil and garlic. Place in an even layer on the baking tray.

2.   Roast broccoli in the oven for 25 minutes or until tender.

3.   Heat remaining oil in a medium skillet over medium heat. Add zucchini, red pepper flakes, onion and parsley. Cook 5 minutes then add the lentils, salt, pepper and broccoli mixture from the oven. Continuously stir for 1 minute.

4.   Garnish with nutritional yeast and serve warm.

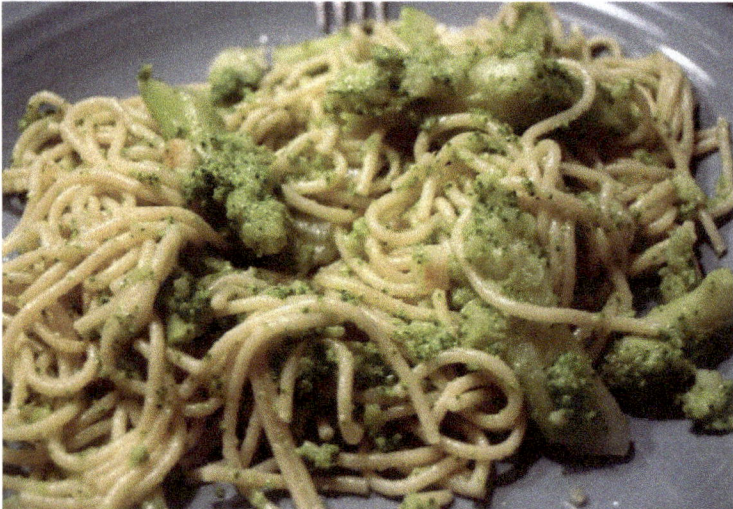

Roasted Vegetable, Hummus & Quinoa Bake

Servings: 2

Total Time: 40 minutes

Ingredients

- 1 cup fresh tomatoes, diced
- 3 shallots, sliced
- 2 small zucchinis, cubed
- 1 cup broccoli, florets cut into small pieces
- 1 yellow bell pepper, chopped
- 2 garlic cloves, minced
- 2 tablespoons coconut oil
- ½ teaspoon Himalayan salt
- ½ teaspoon black pepper, crushed
- ½ teaspoon turmeric
- 1 tablespoon parsley
- 1 cup quinoa, cooked
- 1 ½ cups hummus
- 2 tablespoons nutritional yeast

Directions

1.   Preheat oven to 400°F/205°C. Line a baking tray with parchment paper. In a medium bowl, toss tomatoes, shallots, zucchini, broccoli, bell pepper and garlic with 1 ½ tablespoons coconut oil, salt, pepper and turmeric. Place on the baking tray in an even layer and roast in the oven for 25 minutes or until tender.

2.   In a small bowl, combine the parsley and quinoa.

3.   Grease a small glass baking dish with the remaining ½ tablespoon coconut oil. Place quinoa in a single layer on the bottom of the dish. Spread a layer of hummus on top of the quinoa. Top with roasted vegetables.

4.   Sprinkle with nutritional yeast and bake in the oven for 10 minutes.

5.   Remove and serve immediately.

Spicy Pepper Soup

Servings: 2

Total Time: 55 minutes

Ingredients

- 1 yellow squash, diced
- ¼ red bell pepper, chopped
- 1 shallot, sliced
- 1 tablespoon coconut oil
- ½ 15 ounce can coconut milk
- 2 teaspoons red curry paste
- ½ teaspoon turmeric powder
- 1 lime, juiced
- ½ teaspoon Himalayan salt
- 1 cup brown rice, cooked
- 1 tablespoon cilantro, chopped
- 1 tablespoon cashews, toasted

Directions

1.   Preheat oven to 375°F/190°C. Line a baking tray with parchment paper. Toss squash, bell pepper and shallot with coconut oil in a medium bowl. Place on the baking tray in an even layer. Roast in the oven for 30 minutes or until tender.

2.   In a medium saucepan, heat coconut milk, curry paste and turmeric over medium heat until red curry paste is completely dissolved, about 8 minutes.

3.   Remove vegetables from the oven and let cool for 5 minutes. Then, add to a food processor along with the coconut milk/curry mixture, lime juice and salt. Blend until smooth.

4.   Return to the medium saucepan and bring to a boil. Reduce heat to low and simmer 10 minutes.

5.   Serve along with brown rice and garnish with cilantro and cashews.

Rainbow Spaghetti Squash

Servings: 2

Total Time: 30 minutes

Ingredients

- 2 tablespoons coconut oil, divided
- 1 spaghetti squash, halved lengthwise and seeds removed
- ½ red onion, thinly sliced
- 1 orange bell pepper, sliced
- 1 cup red cabbage, thinly sliced
- 2 green onions, sliced
- 1 cup kale, stems removed and thinly sliced
- 1 cup quinoa, quinoa
- 2 teaspoon dried thyme
- 1 teaspoon oregano
- 1 teaspoon garlic powder
- ½ teaspoon Himalayan salt
- ½ teaspoon black pepper, crushed
- 1 tablespoon pine nuts, toasted
- 1 tablespoon parsley, chopped

- 1 tablespoon nutritional yeast

Directions

1.   Preheat oven to 400°F/205°C. Line a baking tray with parchment paper. Brush 1 tablespoon of oil on the cut sides of the squash and place cut side down on the baking tray.

2.   Roast in the oven for 25 minutes or until tender.

3.   While squash cooks, add remaining oil to a medium saucepan and add onion, bell pepper, cabbage and green onions. Cook 8 minutes until vegetables are softened. Stir in kale and cook another 3 minutes. Add quinoa, thyme, oregano, garlic powder, salt and pepper. Cook 2 more minutes and turn off the heat.

4.   Remove the squash from the oven and, with a fork, loosen some of the flesh of the squash. Spoon half the quinoa and vegetable mixture into each squash half.

5.   Garnish with pine nuts, parsley and nutritional yeast before serving.

Sweet Tofu & Vegetables

Servings: 2

Total Time: 25 minutes

Ingredients

- 1 tablespoon coconut oil

- ½ cup carrot, sliced

- 2 shallots, sliced

- 1 cup red cabbage, thinly shredded

- ½ cup red bell pepper, seeded, and sliced

- 2 cups broccoli, cut into florets

- ¼ teaspoon red chili flakes

- 6 ounces tofu, cubed and baked

- ½ cup cashews, chopped

- 1 tablespoon cilantro, chopped

Sauce

- ½ tablespoon arrowroot powder

- ½ tablespoon roughly chopped fresh ginger

- 2 garlic cloves

- ¼ cup water

- 2 tablespoons tamari
- 1 tablespoon coconut aminos
- 1 tablespoon maple syrup
- ¼ tablespoon lime juice
- 1 tablespoon cilantro

Directions

1.   Prepare the Sauce by adding all the Sauce ingredients to a blender and mixing until smooth. Set aside.

2.   Heat coconut oil in a medium skillet over medium-high heat and add carrot, shallot, cabbage, bell pepper and broccoli. Sauté for 10 minutes and then add chili flakes and tofu. Cook another 5 minutes before adding the Sauce.

3.   Lower heat to low and let Sauce come to a light simmer. Add cashews and cook for another 2 minutes.

4.   Garnish with cilantro before serving.

Lime Green Pasta

Servings: 2

Total Time: 10 minutes

Ingredients

- 2 zucchinis, spiralized
- 1 cup edamame, shelled and cooked
- 2 tablespoons green onions
- 1 green bell pepper, seeded and thinly sliced
- 1 cup green cabbage, thinly shredded

Lime Sauce

- 1 ripe avocado, pit and skin removed
- ½ cup spinach
- ¼ cup fresh cilantro
- 1 lime, juiced
- ½ cup water
- 1 teaspoon raw honey
- ½ teaspoon tamari
- ¼ teaspoon coconut aminos
- ¼ teaspoon Himalayan salt

- ¼ teaspoon black pepper, crushed

- ¼ teaspoon cayenne

Directions

1.   Prepare the Lime Sauce by adding all the Lime Sauce ingredients to a blender and processing until smooth. Set aside.

2.   In a large bowl, combine the zucchini, edamame, green onions, bell pepper and cabbage. Pour Lime Sauce on top and toss until well coated.

3.   Serve immediately.

Roasted Eggplant & Quinoa

Servings: 2

Total Time: 30 minutes plus 1 hour of resting

Ingredients

- 2 small eggplants, cut into cubes
- ¾ teaspoon Himalayan salt
- 1 tablespoon olive oil
- ¼ teaspoon dried thyme
- ¼ teaspoon dried oregano
- 2 tablespoons sesame seeds
- 1 cup quinoa, cooked
- 1 cup arugula
- ¼ cup pine nuts, toasted
- ¼ cup golden raisins
- ¼ teaspoon nutmeg
- ½ cup parsley, chopped
- ¼ cup mint, chopped
- 1 lemon, zested and juiced

Directions

1.   Place eggplant cubes in a colander in the sink or over a bowl. Sprinkle with ½ teaspoon of salt and let sit for 1 hour. Rinse and pat dry.

2.   Preheat oven to 400°F/205°C and line a baking tray with parchment paper. In a medium bowl, combine the eggplant, olive oil, thyme, oregano, ¼ teaspoon salt and sesame seeds. Place eggplant on baking tray and roast in the oven for 20 minutes, flipping once halfway through.

3.   In a large bowl, combine the roasted eggplant, quinoa, arugula, pine nuts, raisins, nutmeg, parsley, mint and lemon juice.

4.   Garnish with lemon zest and serve immediately.

Minted Fruit Salad

Servings: 2

Total Time: 20 minutes

Ingredients

- 2 teaspoons raw honey
- 1 lime, juiced
- 1 tablespoon fresh mint, chopped
- Pinch Himalayan salt
- ½ cup raspberries
- ½ cup blackberries
- 1/3 cup blueberries
- ½ cup pineapple, diced

Directions

1. In a small bowl mix together the honey, lime juice, mint and pinch of salt.

2. In a large bowl combine the raspberries, blackberries, blueberries and pineapple.

3. Pour the honey mint mixture over the fruit and toss to combine. Let sit for 15 minutes before serving.

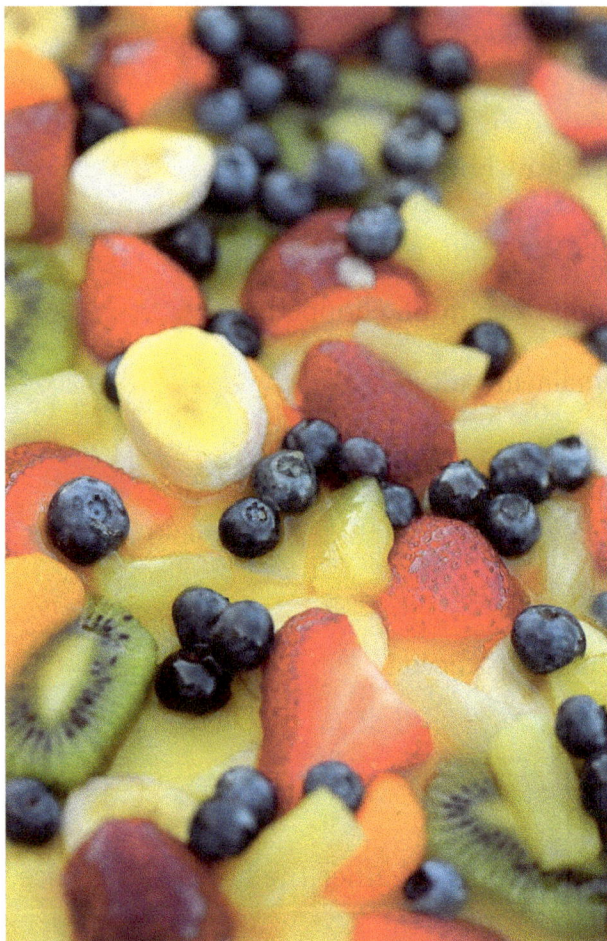

Apricot Tarts

Servings: Makes 8 tarts

Total Time: 30 minutes

Ingredients

- ½ cup raw almonds
- ¾ cup dried dates, pitted and soaked for 15 minutes
- 1 teaspoon nutmeg
- 1 teaspoon cinnamon
- ½ teaspoon Himalayan salt
- 2 small apricots, sliced into 16 pieces
- 8 small mint leaves

Cashew Filling

- ½ cup raw cashews, soaked for 1 hour and drained
- 3 tablespoons lemon juice
- ½ tablespoon lemon zest
- 3 tablespoons water
- 1 teaspoon vanilla extract
- 1 teaspoon raw honey
- ½ teaspoon Himalayan salt

Directions

1.   Make tarts shell dough by combining the almonds, drained dates, nutmeg, cinnamon and salt in a food processor. Pulse until mixture becomes crumbly then continue to blend until a slightly sticky ball forms.

2.   Remove tart shell dough from food processor and form into 8 equal sized balls. Press down each ball into a mini muffin or tart pan, making sure to create equal sides. Place pan in fridge for 10 minutes and then remove the shells.

3.   In a clean food processor, combine the Cashew Filling ingredients until smooth. Place in a bowl and let chill for 10 minutes.

4.   In each tart shell, add the Cashew Filling and top with two apricot slices and a mint leaf.

Sweet Potato Tarts

Servings: Makes 8 tarts

Total Time: 40 minutes

Ingredients

- ½ cup raw almonds
- ¾ cup dried dates, pitted and soaked for 15 minutes
- 1 teaspoon nutmeg
- 1 teaspoon cinnamon
- ½ teaspoon Himalayan salt

Sweet Potato Filling

- 2 small sweet potatoes, peeled and cut into large cubes
- ¼ cup unsweetened almond milk
- 1 teaspoon nutmeg
- 1 teaspoon cinnamon
- ½ teaspoon vanilla extract

Whipped Coconut Cream (optional)

- 1 can full fat coconut milk, chilled overnight in the fridge
- ½ teaspoon vanilla extract
- ½ teaspoon lemon zest

- 1 tablespoon maple syrup

Directions

1.   Make tarts shell dough by combining the almonds, drained dates, nutmeg, cinnamon and salt in a food processor. Pulse until mixture becomes crumbly then continue to blend until a slightly sticky ball forms.

2.   Remove tart shell dough from food processor and form into 8 equal sized balls. Press down each ball into a mini muffin or tart pan, making sure to create equal sides. Place pan in fridge for 10 minutes and then remove the shells.

3.   Place sweet potato in a medium saucepan and cover with water. Bring to a boil over medium heat and then reduce heat to low and simmer for 15 minutes or until sweet potatoes are soft.

4.   Transfer sweet potatoes to the food processor and add almond milk, nutmeg, cinnamon and vanilla extract. Blend until smooth and chill for 10 minutes.

5.   If using the Whipped Coconut Cream, open the can of coconut milk and drain the water for later use. Add coconut cream to a bowl (preferably a chilled metal bowl) and add the vanilla, zest and maple syrup. Beat with a hand mixer for 3 minutes or until fluffy.

6. In each tart shell, add the Sweet Potato Filling and top with the Whipped Coconut Cream. Chill before serving.

Creamy Tropical Ice Pops

Servings: Makes 4 popsicles

Total Time: 5 minutes plus 8 hours of freeze time

Ingredients

- ½ cup pineapple, cubed (not frozen)

- ½ banana

- ½ cup cashews, soaked overnight and drained

- 1 cup unsweetened coconut milk (from can)

- 2 dates, pitted, soaked 15 minutes and drained

- ½ teaspoon vanilla extract

- 1 teaspoon raw honey

Directions

1.   Blend all ingredients in a high speed blender.

2.   Pour mixture into 4 ice pop molds. Halfway through freezing, insert popsicle sticks.

3.   Freeze for a total of 8 hours.

Nutty Oatmeal Raisin Cookies

Servings: Makes 12 cookies

Total Time: 25 minutes

Ingredients

- 1 cup spelt flour
- ½ teaspoon baking soda
- ½ teaspoon salt
- 1 cup gluten free rolled oats
- 1/3 cup almond butter, melted
- 2 tablespoons olive oil
- 1 cup coconut sugar
- 1/3 cup unsweetened almond milk
- 1 teaspoon vanilla extract
- ¼ cup raisins
- ¼ cup walnuts
- ½ cup slivered almonds
- 2 tablespoons dried currants

Directions

1.   Preheat oven to 400°F/205°C. Prepare baking tray by lining with parchment paper.

2.   In a small bowl, sift together the flour, baking soda and salt. Stir in oats.

3.   In a large bowl whisk together the almond butter, olive oil, coconut sugar, almond milk and vanilla extract.

4.   Add dry ingredients to the wet ingredients and stir well to combine. Mix in the raisins, walnuts, almonds and currants.

5.   Drop spoonfuls of the cookie dough on baking tray. Bake for approximately 8 - 10 minutes or until cookies start to brown. Cool completely before serving.

Raspberry & Chocolate Mousse Jars

Servings: 2

Total Time: 15 minutes

Ingredients

- 1 large ripe avocado

- 1/3 cup raw cacao powder

- ¼ cup almond milk

- 3 - 4 dates, pitted, soaked for 15 minutes and drained

- 1 teaspoon vanilla extract

- ¾ cup fresh raspberries

- ¼ teaspoon Himalayan salt

- 1 teaspoon maple syrup (optional)

- 2 tablespoon almond slivers, toasted

- 2 small mint leaves

Directions

1. In a food processor, puree the avocado until smooth. Add in cacao, almond milk, dates, and vanilla extract. Continue to mix until very smooth and well combined.

2.   Add ½ raspberries and salt to the avocado mixture and continue to process in the food processor. Taste and if more sweetness is desired, add in maple syrup.

3.   Spoon mixture into 2 jars and top each with the rest of the raspberries, almond slivers and a mint leaf. Chill 5 minutes before serving.

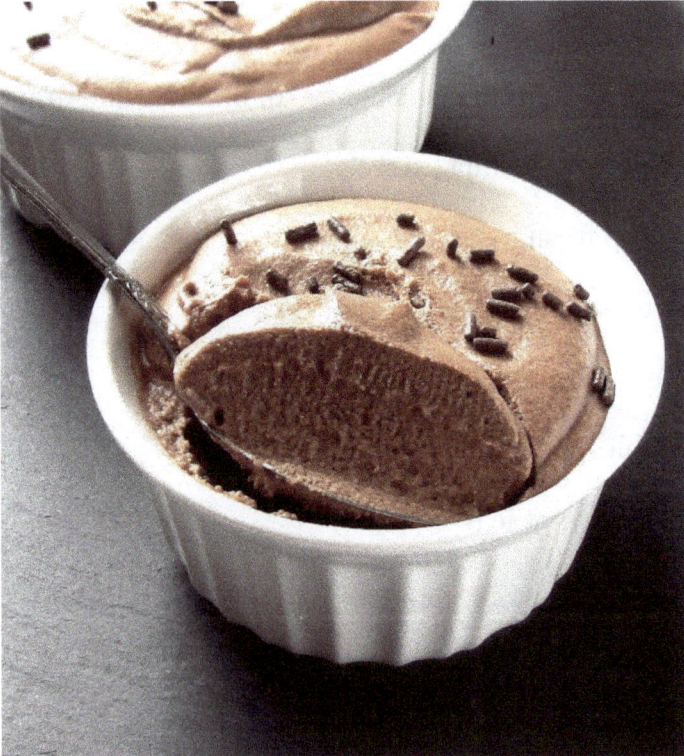

Refreshing Fruit & Cilantro Pops

Servings: Makes 4 popsicles

Total Time: 5 minutes plus 8 hours freeze time

Ingredients

- ½ cup pineapple cubes
- ½ cup mango cubes
- 2 tablespoons cilantro
- 1 tablespoon lime juice
- ½ banana
- 1 tablespoon raw honey
- ¾ cup coconut water

Directions

1. Blend all ingredients together in a blender until smooth.

2. Pour into ice pop molds and place in freezer. Halfway through insert popsicle sticks.

3. Freeze for a total of 8 hours.

Lemon Pudding & Raspberry Tarts

Servings: Makes 8 tarts

Total Time: 30 minutes

Ingredients

- ½ cup raw almonds

- ¾ cup dried dates, pitted and soaked for 15 minutes

- 1 teaspoon lemon zest

- ½ teaspoon Himalayan salt

- 8 fresh raspberries

- 8 small mint leaves

Lemon Pudding

- 2 ½ lemons, juiced

- ¾ cup almond milk

- 3 egg yolks

- 3 ½ tablespoons cornstarch

- ¼ teaspoon Himalayan salt

- 1 cup water

- 1/3 cup raw honey

Directions

1.   Make Lemon Pudding by placing a medium saucepan over medium-low heat and whisking in the lemon juice, almond milk and egg yolks. Continue stirring until mixture comes to a boil. Turn heat off.

2.   Mix together the cornstarch, salt and water. Stir into lemon and egg mixture then stir in the honey.

3.   Make tarts shell dough by combining the almonds, drained dates, lemon zest and salt in a food processor. Pulse until mixture becomes crumbly then continue to blend until a slightly sticky ball forms.

4.   Remove tart shell dough from food processor and form into 8 equal sized balls. Press each ball into a mini muffin or tart pan, making sure to create equal sides. Place pan in fridge for 10 minutes and then remove the shells.

5.   Spoon Lemon Pudding into each tart shell. Top each with a raspberry and mint leaf.

Coconut Cashew Figs

Servings: Makes 10 figs

Total Time: 10 minutes

Ingredients

- 10 dried figs, pitted and split in half
- 10 teaspoons cashew butter
- ¼ cup shredded or ground coconut
- ½ teaspoon cinnamon
- ½ teaspoon nutmeg
- ¼ teaspoon Himalayan salt

Directions

1. Stuff each fig with 1 teaspoon cashew butter and close two sides together as much as possible.

2. On a small plate, combine the coconut, cinnamon, nutmeg and salt. Roll each fig into the coconut mixture and serve.

Cabbage Rolls

Servings: 2

Total Time: 2 hours 10 minutes

Ingredients

- ½ cup brown rice, cooked
- 1 celery stalk, finely diced
- 1 carrot, finely diced
- ½ red bell pepper, finely diced
- ½ teaspoon Himalayan salt
- ½ teaspoon garlic powder
- ½ teaspoon onion powder
- 1 teaspoon parsley, chopped
- 2 tablespoons tomato paste
- 4 cups water
- 8 cabbage leaves
- 2 cups vegetable broth

Directions

1.   Prepare vegetable filling combining brown rice, celery, carrots, red bell pepper, salt, garlic powder, onion powder, parsley and tomato paste in a medium bowl. Set aside in the fridge until ready to use.

2.   In a large pot, bring 4 cups water to a boil. Add cabbage leaves for 1 minute then turn heat off and let sit, covered, for 1 hour.

3.   Remove cabbage leaves from the pot and discard water. Spoon vegetable and rice mixture into each of the cabbage leaves. Roll each cabbage leaf, ensuring there are no openings and secure with a toothpick.

4.   Add vegetable broth to the large pot and lay cabbage rolls on the bottom, toothpick side down. Turn heat to low and simmer for 1 hour.

Lentil Stuffed Squash

Servings: 2

Total Time: 30 minutes

Ingredients

- 1 tablespoon olive oil
- ½ cup red bell pepper, finely diced
- ½ cup zucchini, finely diced
- 1 shallot, diced
- 1 garlic clove, minced
- 2 small acorn squash, halved and seeded
- Non-Stick Vegetable Spray
- ½ cup brown lentils, cooked
- ½ cup quinoa, cooked
- 2 tablespoons coconut aminos

Directions

1. Preheat oven to 350°F/180°C.

2. In a small skillet over medium heat, add olive oil, bell pepper, zucchini, shallot and garlic. Cook 5 minutes and set aside.

3.   Place acorn squash in a medium baking dish sprayed with Non-Stick Vegetable Spray and pour water into the pan so that is ¼ up the side of the squash. Bake 15 minutes and remove.

4.   In a small bowl, combine the vegetable mixture, brown lentils, quinoa and coconut aminos.

5.   Fill each acorn half with the lentil and vegetable mixture and place back in the oven for 10 minutes.

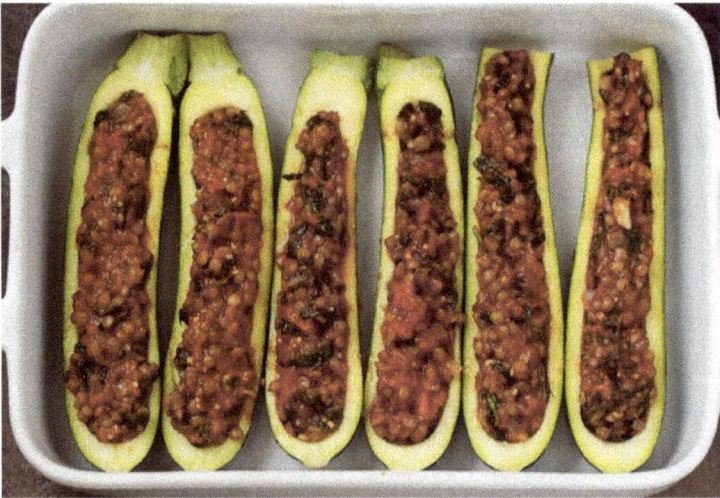

Pomegranate Pumpkins

Servings: 2

Total Time: 35 minutes

Ingredients

- 1 small sugar pumpkin, halved and seeds removed
- 1 tablespoon coconut oil, melted
- ½ cup brown rice, cooked
- ½ cup cooked chickpeas, cooked
- 3 tablespoons pomegranate seeds
- 5 tablespoons parsley, finely chopped
- 1 tablespoon chia seeds
- 1 garlic clove, minced
- 1 teaspoon Himalayan salt
- 1 tablespoon lemon juice
- 1 teaspoon orange juice

Directions

1. Preheat oven to 350°F/180°C.

2.   On a baking tray, place sugar pumpkins and brush with coconut oil. Flip over so that pumpkin is facing down and roast for 25-30 minutes, until flesh is tender.

3.   Once pumpkin is cooked, remove the flesh and place in a large mixing bowl. Add in rice, chickpeas, pomegranate seeds, parsley, chia seeds, garlic, salt, lemon juice and orange juice.

4.   Place mixture back into pumpkin and serve.

Roasted Green Salad

Servings: 2

Total Time: 35 minutes

Ingredients

- 2 cups brussel sprouts, halved
- 1 teaspoon avocado oil
- ¼ teaspoon Himalayan salt
- ¼ teaspoon ground cumin
- 2 teaspoon avocado oil
- 1 garlic clove, minced
- 1 shallot, sliced
- 1 cup green cabbage, shredded
- 1 teaspoon ground oregano
- 1 lemon, zested and juiced
- 1 teaspoon apple cider vinegar
- ½ cup frozen peas, defrosted
- 2 tablespoons chopped mint
- 2 tablespoons almonds, slivered

Directions

1.   Preheat oven to 350°F/180°C.

2.   On a large baking tray, place brussel sprouts, 1 teaspoon avocado oil, salt and cumin. Toss to coat well and roast for 25 minutes.

3.   In a large skillet over medium heat add the other teaspoon of avocado oil, the garlic and shallot. Add the cabbage, oregano, lemon zest and juice and cook for 15 minutes.

4.   Add vinegar and peas to the skillet along with the roasted brussel sprouts and cook for 5 minutes. Transfer to large bowl and toss with the mint and almonds.

Roasted Green Salad

Servings: 2

Total Time: 1 hour

Ingredients

- 4 cups vegetable stock
- 3 tablespoons avocado oil
- 2 garlic cloves, finely minced
- 2 large shallots, finely diced
- 1 cup brown rice
- 2 cups baby spinach, finely chopped
- 1 lemon, zested and juiced
- 1 teaspoon Himalayan salt
- 2 teaspoon black pepper, crushed
- 3 tablespoons green onions, sliced
- 1 cup broccoli sprouts

Directions

1.   In a small saucepan, bring vegetable stock to a low simmer over low heat.

2.   In a large stockpot over medium-low, add avocado oil, garlic and shallot. Cook for 5 minutes before stirring in the brown rice. Stir brown rice for 2 minutes in the pan so that it does not burn. Reduce heat to low.

3.   Add in 1/3 cup of the vegetable stock and stir frequently until the liquid is absorbed. Once liquid is absorbed, add in another 1/3 cup of stock. Continue doing this until all the stock is used and the rice is tender.

4.   While risotto is cooking, add spinach, lemon juice and salt to a blender and combine until smooth.

5.   When risotto is cooked, stir in the spinach mixture and let cook for 3 minutes (rice should absorb most of the spinach liquid).

6.   Stir in lemon zest and black pepper.

7.   Garnish with green onions and broccoli sprouts and serve immediately.

Jumbo Stuffed Mushrooms

Servings: 2

Total Time: 30 minutes

Ingredients

- 2 large Portobello mushrooms
- 2 tablespoons olive oil
- 1 garlic clove, finely minced
- ½ white onion, diced
- ½ cup almonds, slivered and roughly chopped
- 1 cup spinach, chopped
- 2 tablespoons raisins
- ½ teaspoon cinnamon
- ½ teaspoon nutmeg
- 3 tablespoons water
- 3 tablespoons parsley
- 1 teaspoon Himalayan salt
- 1 teaspoon black pepper, crushed.

Directions

1.　　Preheat oven to 350°F/180°C.

2.　　On a large baking tray, place mushrooms, stem side up and drizzle with 1 tablespoon olive oil and the garlic. Roast in the oven for 10 minutes.

3.　　In a large skillet over medium heat add the other tablespoon of olive oil and the onion. Cook for 5 minutes before adding the almonds, spinach, raisins, cinnamon and nutmeg. Let cook for another 4 minutes and then begin adding the water in, one tablespoon at a time and letting the water absorb in between each addition.

4.　　Stir in parsley, salt and pepper before placing the mixture on each of the mushrooms.

5.　　Place back in the oven for another 10 minutes.

Raw Zoodles with Tropical Sauce

Servings: 1

Total Time: 5 minutes

Ingredients

- ½ mango, diced

- ¼ cup pineapple, diced

- 2 tablespoons orange juice

- ½ avocado

- 3 tablespoons green onions, sliced

- 1 garlic clove

- 1 zucchini, spiralized into noodles

Directions

1.   In a blender, combine the mango, pineapple, orange juice, avocado, onions and garlic.

2.   Mix sauce with zucchini noodles and serve.

Spaghetti Squash Pasta Boats

Servings: 2

Total Time: 30 minutes

Ingredients

- 1 spaghetti squash, halved lengthwise and seeds removed
- 2 tablespoons olive oil
- 1 teaspoon Himalayan salt
- 1 teaspoon black pepper, crushed
- 2 garlic cloves, minced
- 5 handfuls kale, stems removed and sliced thinly
- 1 cup of chickpeas, cooked
- ¼ cup raisins
- ¼ cup of walnuts
- 1 avocado, sliced

Directions

1. Preheat oven to 350°F/180°C.

2.   On a large baking tray, brush squash halves with 1 tablespoon olive oil and season with salt and pepper. Place squash cut side down and roast for 25 minutes or until tender.

3.   In a large skillet over medium heat add the other tablespoon of olive oil and the garlic. Cook for 2 minutes before adding the kale, chickpeas, raisins and walnuts. Let cook for another 8 minutes.

4.   With a fork, loosen the strands of the squash and then pour in the kale and chickpea mixture.

5.   Top with avocado slices.

Sweet Potato Chili

Servings: 2

Total Time: 45 minutes

Ingredients

- 1 tablespoon coconut oil
- 2 garlic cloves, minced
- ½ yellow onion, diced
- ½ inch knob ginger, minced
- 1 tablespoon turmeric
- ½ teaspoon coriander
- ¼ teaspoon cumin
- ¼ teaspoon cinnamon
- 2 small sweet potatoes, chopped into small chunks
- 1 large tomato, diced
- ½ cup red lentils
- ½ cup quinoa
- 1 15-ounce can tomato puree
- 2 cups water
- 1 bunch kale, stems removed and chopped into pieces

- 1 lemon, juiced

- 1 teaspoon Himalayan salt

- 2 tablespoons green onions, sliced

- 1 tablespoon cashews, chopped

Directions

1.   Heat coconut oil in a large pot over medium heat. Add garlic, onion, ginger, turmeric, coriander, cumin and cinnamon. Cook for 5 minutes and then add sweet potato and let cook for another 5 minutes.

2.   Stir in diced tomato, red lentils, quinoa, tomato puree and water. Bring to a boil, reduce heat to low and let simmer for 25 minutes.

3.   Stir in kale, lemon juice and salt. Let simmer another 5 minutes.

4.   Transfer to bowl and garnish with green onions and cashews.

Sweet Potato Cottage Platter

Servings: 2

Total Time: 50 minutes

Ingredients

- 2 teaspoons olive oil
- 1 yellow onion, chopped small
- 1 garlic clove, minced
- ½ carrot, diced
- 1 celery stalk, diced
- 5 button mushrooms, sliced
- ½ cup green peas
- 2 tomatoes, diced
- 1 teaspoon cumin powder
- ½ teaspoon turmeric powder
- ½ teaspoon cayenne
- 2 teaspoons tamari sauce
- 1 teaspoon coconut aminos
- ¼ cup tomato paste
- 2 tablespoons water

- 2 bay leaves

- 1 teaspoon chives, sliced

Mashed Topping

- 2 sweet potatoes, peeled and chopped

- 2 cups water

- 1 teaspoon Himalayan salt

- 1 teaspoon nutmeg

- ¼ cup unsweetened almond milk

Directions

1.   In a large saucepan over medium heat, add olive oil, onion, garlic, carrot and celery. Cook for 5 minutes and then add the mushrooms, peas, tomatoes, cumin, turmeric, cayenne, tamari, coconut aminos, tomato paste, water and bay leaves.

2.   Reduce heat to low and simmer for 15 minutes. Remove bay leaves and pour vegetable mixture into a small glass baking dish.

3.   In a medium saucepan, make the Mashed Topping by covering sweet potatoes with water. Bring to a boil and then reduce heat and let simmer for 20 minutes or until sweet potatoes are tender. Drain potatoes and blend in a food processor with salt, nutmeg and almond milk until smooth.

4.   Preheat oven to 350°F/180°C. Place mashed sweet potato on top of the vegetable mixture in the baking dish. Smooth out the top with a knife and bake in the oven for 30 minutes.

5.   Garnish with the chives and serve warm.

Italian Stuffed Zucchini

Servings: 2

Total Time: 50 minutes

Ingredients

- 1 cup cherry tomatoes, halved

- 2 cups spinach, chopped

- 1 tablespoon lemon zest

- ½ teaspoon Himalayan salt

- ½ teaspoon black pepper, crushed

- ½ teaspoon red chili flakes

- 1 garlic clove, grated

- 2 teaspoons pine nuts

- 1 tablespoon olive oil, divided

- 2 large zucchinis, split in half lengthwise and seeds removed

- 1 ½ cup basil, sliced thinly

Directions

1. Preheat oven to 400°F/205°C.

2.   In a small bowl, combine the tomatoes, spinach, zest, salt, black pepper, chili flakes, garlic and pine nuts. Drizzle with half of the olive oil and toss to coat well.

3.   Stuff each half of the zucchini with the cherry and spinach mixture. Place on baking tray and roast in the oven for 15 minutes.

4.   Remove from the oven and drizzle with remaining olive oil and garnish with basil.

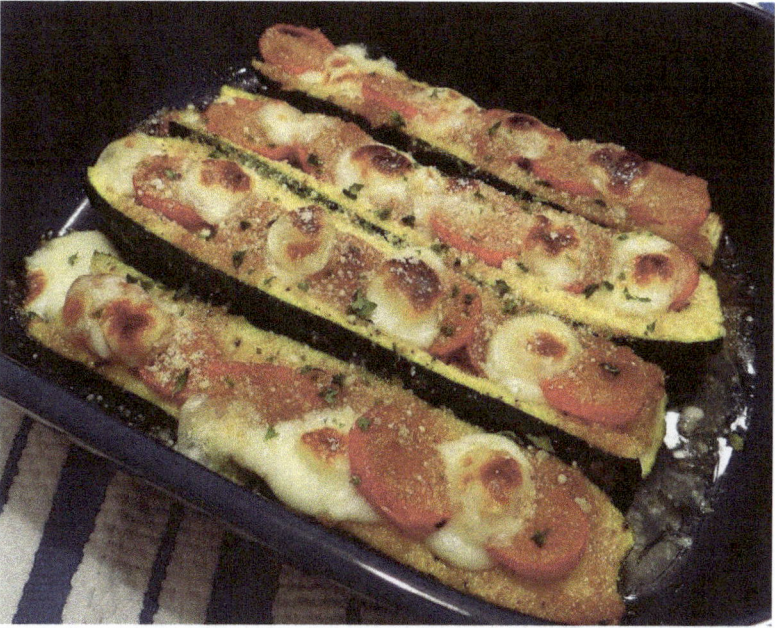

Sushi Bowl

Servings: 2

Total Time: 40 minutes

Ingredients

- ¼ cup tamari
- 2 tablespoons coconut aminos
- 2 teaspoon sesame oil
- 2 tablespoon sesame seeds
- 2 tablespoon chopped shallots
- 1 garlic clove, minced
- 1 ½ inch piece of ginger, grated
- 1 lime, zested and juiced
- 1 jalapeno, seeded and diced
- 2 sashimi grade tuna medallions, cubed
- 1 cup quinoa, cooked
- 2 tablespoons green onions, sliced
- 3 tablespoons cilantro, chopped
- 1 carrot, spiralized
- 1 avocado

Directions

1.   In a medium sized bowl, whisk the tamari, coconut aminos, 1 teaspoon sesame oil, 1 tablespoon sesame seeds, shallots, garlic, ginger, lime zest, lime juice and jalapeno. Place tuna in the bowl and toss to coat. Place in fridge for 30 minutes.

2.   In a separate medium bowl, combine the quinoa, green onions and 1 tablespoon of the cilantro. Place in serving bowls and add spiralized carrot and avocado on one side of each bowl.

3.   Remove tuna from fridge and place next to the carrot and avocado. Garnish with 2 tablespoons cilantro, 1 tablespoon sesame seeds and drizzle with 1 teaspoon sesame oil.

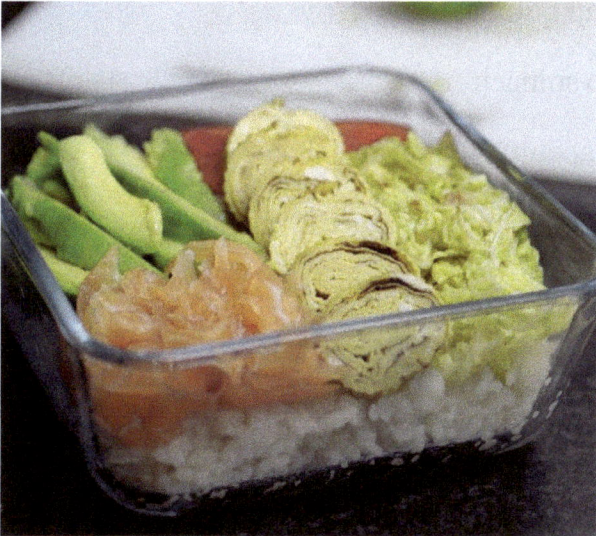

Omega Super Bowl

Servings: 2

Total Time: 25 minutes

Ingredients

- 1 tablespoon ghee
- 1 shallot, sliced
- 1 garlic clove, minced
- ½ head of broccoli, cut into small florets
- 6 ounces salmon fillet
- ½ cup almond milk
- ½ cup quinoa, cooked
- 1 cup spinach
- 1 teaspoon Himalayan salt
- 1 teaspoon black pepper, crushed
- 2 teaspoons red chili flakes
- 2 teaspoons flaxseeds oil

Directions

1. In a medium skillet over medium heat, add ghee, shallot and garlic. Cook 2 minutes and then add the broccoli. Let sauté 8 minutes until broccoli is softened. Remove broccoli and set aside.

2. Place salmon in the same skillet and add almond milk. Bring to a boil, cover the pan and reduce heat. Let simmer for 7 minutes or until fish is cooked through.

3. Set aside salmon and add back to the pan the broccoli, and also add quinoa and spinach. Cook for 3 minutes then season with the salt and pepper. Transfer to serving bowls.

4. Gently flake the salmon and divide among the bowls. Sprinkle with chili flakes, drizzle with flaxseeds oil and serve.

Mediterranean Mushrooms

Servings: 2

Total Time: 20 minutes

Ingredients

- 4 Portobello mushrooms, stems removed.
- 2 tablespoons olive oil
- 1 zucchini diced
- ¼ cup sun dried tomatoes, chopped
- ¼ cup of sun ripened black olives
- 1 ½ cups quinoa, cooked
- 1 handful of parsley leaves, finely chopped
- 1 handful of cilantro, finely chopped
- 1 tablespoon of pine nuts
- 1 tablespoon of lemon juice
- 1 teaspoon dried oregano
- 1 teaspoon Himalayan salt
- 1 teaspoon black pepper, crushed

Directions

1.   Line a baking tray with parchment paper and place mushrooms stems side up. Drizzle with 1 tablespoon olive oil and gently massage into the mushroom. Place under the broiler on high heat and cook 4 minutes and then flip and cook 4 more minutes.

2.   Add 1 tablespoon olive oil to a medium skillet over medium heat along with the zucchini, tomatoes and olives. Cook 5 minutes and then add the quinoa and cook for another 3 minutes. Turn heat off and stir in the parsley, cilantro, pine nuts, lemon juice, oregano, salt and pepper.

3.   Top each mushroom with the vegetable and quinoa mixture and serve warm.

Cauliflower Lettuce Cups

Servings: 2

Total Time: 20 minutes

Ingredients

- ½ cauliflower head, chopped into small pieces
- 1 tablespoon coconut oil
- 1 carrot, grated
- 1 cup mushrooms, diced
- 2 shallots, diced
- 1 garlic clove, finely diced
- 1 inch piece of ginger, grated
- 1 tablespoon coconut aminos
- 1 tablespoon tamari
- 1 lime, juiced
- 1 teaspoon Himalayan salt
- 1 teaspoon red chili flakes
- 6 large romaine lettuce leaves
- 1 tablespoon cilantro, chopped
- 1 tablespoon walnuts, chopped

Directions

1.   Add cauliflower pieces to a food processor and pulse a few times until it forms a rice-like consistency.

2.   Place coconut oil in a medium skillet and heat over medium heat. Add carrot, mushrooms, shallot, garlic and ginger to cook for 8 minutes.

3.   Toss in cauliflower, coconut aminos, tamari, lime juice, salt and chili flakes. Cook another 5 minutes until vegetables are tender.

4.   Spoon mixture into each lettuce leaf and garnish with cilantro and walnuts before serving.

Citrus Stir Fry

Servings: 2

Total Time: 10 minutes

Ingredients

- 1 teaspoon sesame oil
- 1 teaspoon coconut oil
- 1 shallot, sliced
- 1 garlic clove, crushed
- ½ cup carrot, shredded
- ½ red bell pepper, seeds removed and sliced
- 1 cup of bok choy, roughly chopped
- 1 tablespoon lime zest
- 1 lime, juiced
- 1 tablespoon fresh ginger, grated
- 3 tablespoons coconut aminos
- 3 tablespoons tamari
- 2 tablespoons water
- 1 zucchini, spiralized into zoodles
- 2 tablespoons cashews

- 2 tablespoons green onions, sliced

- 2 tablespoons cilantro, chopped

Directions

1. Heat oils in a medium skillet or wok over medium-high heat. Add shallot, garlic, carrot, bell pepper and bok choy. Cook for 3 minutes, stirring frequently.

2. Add lime zest, lime juice, ginger, coconut aminos, tamari and water. Cook another 1 minute and turn off heat.

3. Toss in zoodles and transfer to a serving bowl.

4. Garnish with cashews, green onions and cilantro.

Pineapple Boats

Servings: 2

Total Time: 25 minutes

Ingredients

- 1 teaspoon coconut oil
- 1 baby bok choy, sliced
- 1 large carrot, diced
- 1 red bell pepper, diced
- 1 garlic clove, minced
- 1 inch piece ginger, grated
- ½ teaspoon turmeric
- 1 teaspoon red chili flakes
- ½ teaspoon cayenne
- ½ cup coconut cream
- 1 cup water
- 1 pineapple, halved lengthwise and flesh taken (to form a boat with the skin), flesh diced
- 1 cup kale, stems removed and chopped
- ½ cup raw cashews, crushed

- 1 cup quinoa, cooked

- 1 tablespoon cilantro, chopped

Directions

1. Add coconut oil to a large skillet over medium-high heat. Add bok choy, carrot, bell pepper, garlic and ginger and cook for 6 minutes.

2. Stir in turmeric, chili flakes, cayenne, coconut cream, water and diced pineapple. Reduce heat to medium-low and simmer 8 minutes.

3. Add kale, cashews and quinoa to the skillet and cook 2 minutes.

4. Place vegetable and quinoa mixture in the pineapple skin and garnish with cilantro.

Moroccan Vegetable Stew

Servings: 2

Total Time: 55 minutes

Ingredients

- 1 tablespoon olive oil
- ½ cup red onion, chopped
- 1 garlic clove, minced
- 1 carrot, chopped
- 1 sweet potatoes, chopped
- ½ teaspoon coriander
- ½ teaspoon cardamom
- ¼ teaspoon turmeric
- 1 tablespoon fresh ginger root, minced
- 1 large eggplant, chopped
- ½ cup cauliflower, chopped
- ¾ cup vegetable stock
- 1 ½ tablespoon tomato paste
- 1 tablespoon parsley, chopped
- 2 tablespoons mint, chopped

- 1 teaspoon Himalayan salt

- ¼ teaspoon black pepper

- 1 tablespoon lemon zest

- 6-8 green olives

Directions

1.   In a large stockpot add the olive oil, red onion, garlic and carrots over medium heat. Cook for 5 minutes and then add the sweet potatoes, coriander, cardamom, turmeric and ginger root. Toss well to coat and cook another 2 minutes.

2.   Add vegetable stock and tomato paste. Bring to a boil and then reduce heat to low and simmer with the lid on for 40 minutes.

3.   Stir in eggplant, cauliflower, parsley, 1 tablespoon mint, salt, pepper, lemon zest and green olives. Cook an additional 3 minutes and then transfer to serving bowls.

4.   Garnish with remaining tablespoon mint.

Quinoa Stuffed Peppers

Servings: 2

Total Time: 25 minutes

Ingredients

- 2 bell peppers, halved and seeded
- Pinch of Himalayan salt
- 1 teaspoon olive oil
- 1 onion, diced
- 1 garlic clove, minced
- 1 zucchini, diced
- 3 mushrooms, diced
- 1 tomato, diced
- 1 tablespoon dried oregano
- ½ teaspoon dried basil
- ½ teaspoon red chili flakes
- 1 cup quinoa, cooked
- ½ cup fresh parsley, chopped

Directions

1.   Place bell peppers on a baking tray, cut side down, and sprinkle with salt. Place sheet under the broiler on high for 8 minutes or until browned. Flip and cook another 5 minutes.

2.   Heat olive oil in a medium skillet over medium-low heat. Add onion, garlic, zucchini and mushrooms. Cook 5 minutes and then add tomato, oregano, basil and chili flakes. Cook for an additional 5 minutes.

3.   Stir in quinoa and parsley and remove from heat.

4.   Stuff each half of pepper with the quinoa vegetable mixture and place back in the broiler on a baking tray for 6-8 minutes.

5.   Serve and enjoy!

Everything Sweet Potato Pizza

Servings: 2

Total Time: 1 hour 15 minutes

Ingredients

- 2 large sweet potatoes
- 1 garlic clove, minced
- 1 ½ tablespoons coconut oil, melted
- 1 tablespoon chia seeds
- 3 tablespoons water
- 1 ¼ cups gluten free oat flour
- ½ cup almond flour
- 1 tablespoon apple cider vinegar
- 1 teaspoon Himalayan salt
- 1 cup cherry tomatoes, halved
- 1 tablespoon sun dried tomatoes, chopped
- ½ cup black olives, sliced
- 2 tablespoons green onions
- 1 tablespoon nutritional yeast

Spinach Pesto

- 3 cups spinach

- 1 cup basil

- 3 tablespoons olive oil

- 2 garlic cloves

- 1 teaspoon pine nuts

- 1 teaspoon nutritional yeast

- 1 teaspoon Himalayan salt

Directions

1.   Poke holes in the sweet potatoes with a fork and place on a baking tray. Coat with garlic and ½ tablespoon coconut oil.

2.   Roast in an oven that has been preheated to 400°F/205°C for 40 minutes or until sweet potatoes are tender. Remove from oven and scoop flesh out of each sweet potato and place in a bowl.

3.   Whisk together the chia and water in a small bowl and set aside for 10 minutes

4.   Add oat flour, almond flour, remaining coconut oil, vinegar and salt to the sweet potato mixture and stir to combine. Whisk in chia mixture and combine well.

5.   On a baking tray lined with parchment paper, form sweet potato dough into a pizza shape. Place in oven and bake for 30 minutes.

6.   While pizza cooks, add spinach, basil, olive oil, pine nuts, garlic, salt and nutritional yeast to a food processor or blender. Mix until smooth, adding some more olive oil if necessary to thin out the Spinach Pesto.

7.   Once pizza crust is cooked, spread Spinach Pesto on the crust. Top with cherry tomatoes, sun dried tomatoes, olives and green onions. Sprinkle with nutritional yeast and serve.

Lentil Sweet Potato Tacos

Servings: 2

Total Time: 50 minutes

Ingredients

- 2 medium sweet potatoes
- 1 teaspoon avocado oil
- 1 shallot, sliced
- 1 cup lentils, cooked
- 1 teaspoon cumin
- 1 teaspoon chili powder
- ¼ cup green onion, chopped
- 1 teaspoon lime juice
- 1 teaspoon Himalayan salt
- ¼ cup tomatoes, chopped
- 1 avocado, sliced
- 2 teaspoons unsweetened yogurt
- 1 tablespoon cilantro, chopped

Directions

1.   Poke sweet potatoes with a fork several times and roast in the oven at 400°F/205°C for 40 minutes.

2.   While sweet potato cooks, heat oil in a small skillet over medium heat and add shallot, lentils, cumin and chili powder. Cook 5 minutes and then add green onion, lime juice and salt.

3.   When sweet potatoes are cooked, make a 2 inch slit in the top of each and open them up. Spoon lentil mixture into each sweet potato and top with tomatoes, avocado, yogurt and cilantro.

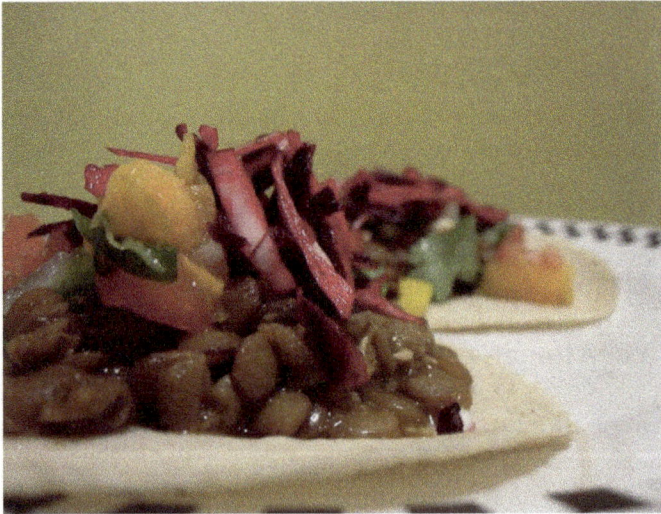

Spaghetti Squash and Meatless Meatballs

Servings: 2

Total Time: 1 hour 5 minutes

Ingredients

- 1 teaspoon olive oil
- 1 spaghetti squash, halved lengthwise and seeds removed
- 1 tablespoon ground flaxseeds
- 3 tablespoons water
- 1 tablespoon coconut oil
- 1 garlic clove, minced
- ½ yellow onion, diced
- ½ cup spinach, chopped
- 1 teaspoon apple cider vinegar
- 1 tablespoon fresh thyme, chopped
- 1 tablespoon fresh parsley, chopped
- 1 teaspoon dried oregano
- 1 teaspoon Himalayan salt
- 1 teaspoon black pepper, crushed
- ½ cup lentils, cooked

- 4 ounces baby bella mushrooms, diced

- ¼ cup quinoa, cooked

- 1 tablespoon almond meal

- ½ cup diced tomatoes

Directions

1. Preheat oven to 400°F/205°C. Rub olive oil on the flesh side of the squash and on a baking tray lined with parchment paper, place squash cut side down. Roast for 30 minutes or until flesh is tender.

2. In a small bowl, whisk together the flaxseeds with 3 tablespoons water. Set aside.

3. Heat coconut oil in a small skillet over medium heat and add garlic and onions. Cook 5 minutes and then add spinach, sautéing another 2 minutes. Add vinegar, thyme, parsley, oregano, salt and pepper. Remove from heat

4. In a food processor, blend lentils and mushrooms until combined. Transfer to a medium bowl and add quinoa, almond meal as well as the mixture from the small skillet and flax mixture. Combine with your hands until you can form balls. Form dough into balls and place on a baking tray. Bake in oven for 30 minutes.

5.   With a fork, remove the flesh from the skin of the squash. Toss in diced tomatoes. Place back in the oven for 10 minutes or until warmed.

6.   Top with lentil mushroom balls and serve.

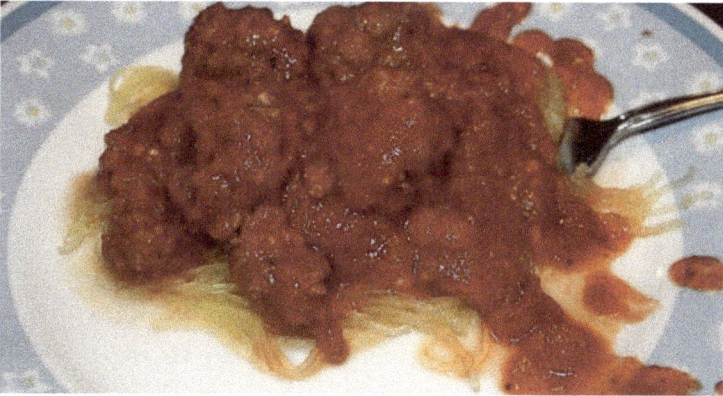

Raw Thai Wraps

Servings: 2

Total Time: 10 minutes

Ingredients

- ½ zucchini, spiralized into thin noodles

- 1 carrot, shredded

- ½ cup red onion, thinly sliced

- ½ cup scallion, sliced

- ½ bunch kale, stems removed and thinly sliced

- ¼ cup red cabbage, shredded

- 2 tablespoons sesame seeds

- 1 teaspoon Himalayan salt

- 1 teaspoon avocado oil

- 1 teaspoon lemon juice

- 3-4 big romaine leaves

Peanut Sauce

- 1 tablespoon of sesame oil

- 1 tablespoon apple cider vinegar

- 2 tablespoons natural peanut butter

- 1 teaspoon coconut aminos

- 1 teaspoon lime juice

- 1 teaspoon cilantro, chopped

Directions

1. In a medium sized bowl, combine zucchini noodles, carrot, red onion, scallion, kale, cabbage, sesame seeds, salt, avocado oil and lemon juice. Toss well and let sit for 5 minutes in the fridge.

2. Make the Peanut Sauce by whisking together the sesame oil, vinegar, peanut butter, coconut aminos, lime juice and cilantro in a small bowl.

3. Place romaine leaves on a platter and spoon the vegetable mixture evenly into each one.

4. Drizzle sauce over each wrap and serve immediately.

Eggplant & Chickpea Stew

Servings: 2

Total Time: 30 minutes

Ingredients

- 1 large eggplant, halved
- 1 teaspoon olive oil, divided
- 1 cup yellow onion, finely diced
- 2 cups tomatoes, diced
- ½ teaspoon fresh ginger, grated
- ½ teaspoon fresh garlic, grated
- ½ teaspoon coriander powder
- 1 teaspoon cumin powder
- ⅛ teaspoon turmeric
- ¼ teaspoon cinnamon
- ½ teaspoon red chili flakes
- 2 tablespoons water
- ¼ teaspoon Himalayan salt
- 1 cup chickpeas, cooked
- 2 tablespoons cilantro, chopped

Directions

1.   Preheat oven to 375°F/190°C. Line a baking tray with parchment paper.

2.   Place eggplant, cut side down, on the baking tray and roast for 20 minutes.

3.   In a large skillet heat olive oil over medium-low heat. Add onion and cook for 5 minutes. Stir in the tomatoes, ginger, garlic, coriander, cumin, turmeric, cinnamon, chili flakes water and salt. Cook for another 5 minutes before adding the chickpeas.

4.   Remove eggplant from the oven, remove the skin and chop into pieces. Toss eggplant into the large skillet with the tomato, spice and chickpea mixture.

5.   Cook for 2 minutes and then transfer to serving bowl and garnish with cilantro.

www.ingramcontent.com/pod-product-compliance
Lightning Source LLC
Chambersburg PA
CBHW050747030426
42336CB00012B/1699